Menopause

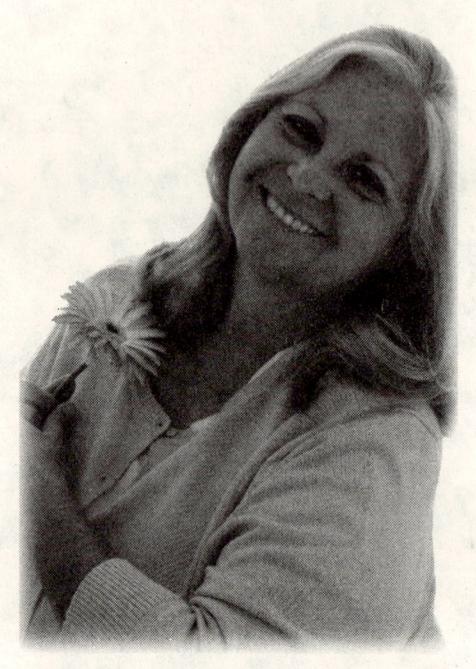

Health Solutions
Menopause

Edited by
Dr Savitri Ramaiah

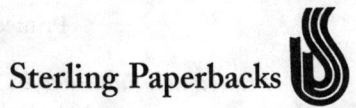
Sterling Paperbacks

STERLING PAPERBACKS
An imprint of
Sterling Publishers (P) Ltd.
A-59, Okhla Industrial Area, Phase-II,
New Delhi-110020.
Tel: 26387070, 26386209; Fax: 91-11-26383788
E-mail: mail@sterlingpublishers.com
www.sterlingpublishers.com

Menopause
© 2008, Sterling Publishers (P) Ltd.
ISBN 978 81 207 3331 2
Reprint 2010, 2011

All rights are reserved.
No part of this publication may be reproduced, stored in a retrieval system or transmitted, in any form or by any means, mechanical, photocopying, recording or otherwise, without prior written permission of the original publisher.

Printed in India

Printed and Published by Sterling Publishers Pvt. Ltd., New Delhi-110 020.

Information for this series, has been provided by *Health Update*, a monthly bulletin of the Society for Health Education and Learning Packages. The Update is intended to provide you with knowledge to adopt preventive measures and cooperate with the doctor during illness for better outcome of treatment.

Contributors

Allopathy
Dr Savitri Ramaiah
(Member-Secretary, HELP and Editor, Health Update)

Ayurveda
Dr V N Pandey
(Former Director, Central Council for Research in Ayurveda and Siddha, New Delhi)

Homoeopathy
Dr Sangeeta Chopra
(Consultant Homoeopathy, New Delhi)

Nature Cure
Dr Sambhashiva Rao
(Consultant, Naturopathy, Pandrapadu, Dist. Guntur, Andhra Pradesh)

Unani
Hakim Mohammed Khalid Siddiqui
(Director, Central Council for Research in Unani, New Delhi)

Preface

Health Solution is an easy-to-read reference series put together by *Health Update* and assisted by a team of medical experts who offer the latest perspectives on body health.

Each book in the series enhances your knowledge on a particular health issue. It makes you an active participant by giving multiple perspectives to choose from — allopathy, acupuncture, ayurveda, homoeopathy, nature cure and unani.

This book is intended as a home adviser but does not substitute a doctor.

The opinions are those of the contributors, and the publisher holds no responsibility.

Contents

Preface	7
Introduction	11
Allopathy	13
Ayurveda	53
Homoeopathy	61
Nature Cure	69
Unani	79
Herbal Extracts	83

Introduction

Menopause is a stage in a woman's life when menstruation stops, thus ending her childbearing years. Although it is a natural process and not a disease, many women approach menopause with an apprehension that they would begin to suffer from several mental and physical conditions. This apprehension is not fully justified. Menopause should and can be the beginning of a positive and satisfying period of your life. It is true that the risk of several health problems increases after menopause but you need to regard it as an opportunity for availing preventive health care for

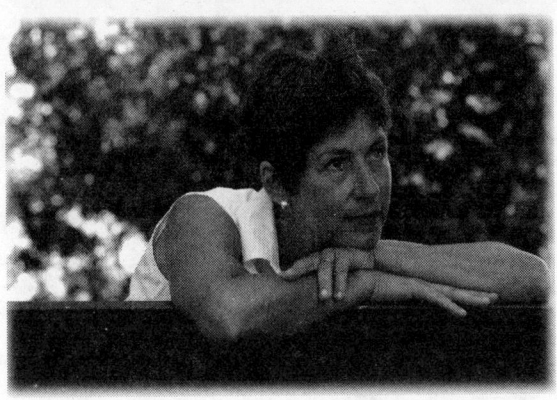

various health problems. These include, among others, controlling body weight, maintaining mental well being and a positive attitude about sexuality, screening for major diseases such as cancer (especially those of reproductive organs), heart diseases, and treatment of disorders of the urinary system.

You are said to have achieved menopause if you have not had a menstrual period for twelve consecutive months and there is no other reason (such as pregnancy, some diseases, etc.) for lack of menstruation. Menopause is the result of loss of the functions of the *ovaries*. Ovaries are female reproductive organs located on each side of the lower abdomen. They produce an egg every month during the reproductive period and secrete the female sex hormones — *estrogen* and *progesterone*.

This issue focuses on the basic facts of menopause, management of some of its troublesome symptoms and its effect on various other organs and systems of the body.

Allopathy

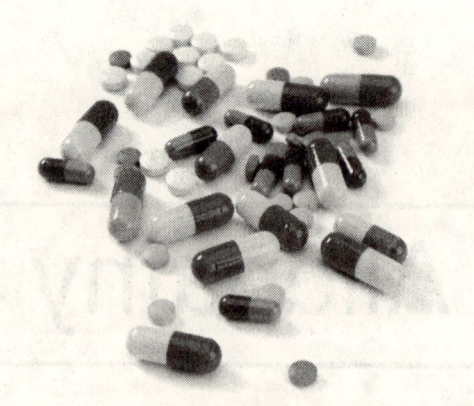

What is the role of estrogen and progesterone in the body?

Estrogen plays a very important role in your body and prepares it for feminine functions such as pregnancy and childbirth. Estrogen and progesterone together regulate the menstrual cycle and the changes that take place in the uterus in preparation for a pregnancy. About ninety per cent of the total estrogen in the body is produced by the ovaries. The remaining amount is produced by other glands such as the liver, adrenal glands and the kidneys. Adrenal glands are secretory organs located on top of each kidney. They produce several hormones, one of which is converted into estrogen in the liver. Fat cells can also make small amounts of estrogen. This is why obese women tend to have less severe symptoms of menopause. However, since obesity is associated with several other health problems, especially heart diseases, you need to maintain normal body weight.

Estrogen stimulates the growth of bones and maintains their normal structure and functions. It also increases the amount of good cholesterol and decreases the amount of bad cholesterol in the blood, thereby protecting the heart and the blood vessels.

Box 1: Functions of female sex hormones

Functions of estrogen:

Reproductive organs:

- Promotes growth and development of reproductive organs of a female such as uterus, vagina, external genital organs, and breasts during puberty.
- Maintains normal structure and functions of the reproductive organs after puberty.

Actions on Uterus:

- Increase the thickness of the uterus by two to three times.
- Increases the blood supply to the uterus.
- Increases the number and length of the glands inside the uterus.
- Promotes secretion of thin watery mucus by the cervix. This watery mucus helps the sperms to move inside the uterus.

Actions on Fallopian tubes:

- Increases the activities of the cells in the fallopian tube. As a result, they secrete more fluids.

- Increases the contractions of the muscles of the fallopian tube. As a result the ovum is easily transported towards the uterus.

Vagina:
- Thickening of the inner lining of the vagina.

Breasts:
- Development of the ducts in the breast that secrete milk after delivery.
- Deposition of fat in the breasts.

Central Nervous System:
- Increases sexual desire.

Bones:
- Increase the rate of bone growth at puberty.

Other actions:
- Lower plasma cholesterol.

Functions of progesterone:
- Progesterone acts only after the action of estrogen on the reproductive organs has taken place.
- In further increases the thickness of the uterus lining and the size of its glands in the second half of the menstrual cycle.
- Ensures continuation of pregnancy.
- Promotes secretion of thick mucus by the cervix after ovulation. It therefore prevents the sperms from entering the uterus.
- Increases body temperature after ovulation.
- Stimulates respiration in the second half of the menstrual cycle and later months of pregnancy.

Progesterone is mainly produced by the ovaries. The adrenal glands produce it in small amounts. It stimulates the growth of the inner lining of the uterus and makes it like a soft cushion where the fertilised egg can grow and develop into a baby. Progesterone plays a very important role in maintaining normal pregnancy. Box 1 lists the major functions of estrogen and progesterone.

What are the types of menopause?

There are two main types of menopause:

- *Natural menopause,* which is due to decrease in the production of female sex hormones — estrogen and progesterone — by the ovaries. It is a gradual process that is normally spread over several years.
- *Induced menopause,* which is due to one of the several medical interventions. For example, surgical removal of both ovaries because of an abnormality in their structure and function before the age of natural menopause causes surgical menopause. Similarly, some medicines, radiation and *chemotherapy* (treatment of various diseases, especially cancer, with chemical agents) can also cause induced menopause. It is a sudden event and this is why the symptoms associated with induced menopause are normally more troublesome.

Induced menopause is not common in women who have had *hysterectomy* before the age of natural menopause. Hysterectomy is the term used for surgical removal of the uterus. Since the ovaries are not removed during this surgery, they can continue to produce sex hormones. However, if the nerves and blood supply to the ovaries are damaged while doing hysterectomy, induced menopause can occur.

When does menopause occur?

Majority of the women experience menopause between the age of forty-five to fifty-five years. Factors that influence the age of menopause include:

Cigarette smoking

This has been identified as one of the major factors that affects the age of menopause. Women who smoke or have been smokers in the past are likely to experience menopause about one and a half to two years earlier.

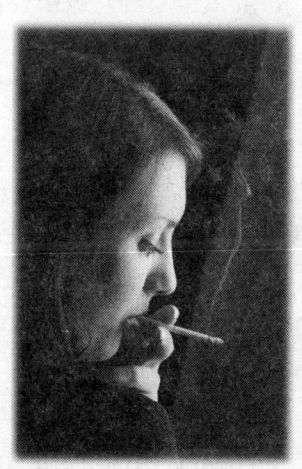

Nutritional status

Women with poor nutritional status experience early menopause.

Body fat
Estrogen production is influenced by the body fat. This is why thin women experience menopause earlier as compared to obese women.

Hereditary
Some studies have indicated that mothers and daughters tend to experience menopause at the same age. However, more studies are needed to determine if genetics is a key factor in determining the age of menopause.

High altitude
Women living in high altitude are more likely to experience early menopause.

Use of oral contraceptives, socio-economic conditions, marriage, height, number of children, and the age of onset of menstruation do not influence the age of menopause.

What are the health problems associated with menopause?

Decrease in functions of the ovaries can have direct and indirect effect on your health. Direct effects include:
- Thinning of the lining of the *vulva* and vagina;
- Urinary problems; and
- Changes in the skin, hair and breasts.

Indirect effects of estrogen deficiency include:
- Hot flushes;
- Loss of bone density; and

- Psychosexual problems.

Some studies have indicated that in addition to the above direct and indirect effects of estrogen deficiency, it may also lead to (a) psychological problems, (b) heart diseases, and (c) changes in the fat metabolism.

What are the symptoms of menopause?

The symptoms of menopause and its severity can vary from woman to woman. Some women do not report any troublesome symptoms while some others report severe symptoms that adversely affect their day-to-day life. Detailed below are some of the common symptoms associated with menopause. These are listed in Box 2.

Irregular bleeding

Most women identify the onset of menopause because of irregular periods. Changes in the menstrual patterns vary from woman to woman. There may be shorter or longer periods, increased or decreased menstrual flow and varying periods of time between two menstrual cycles. You need to consult with your doctor if:

1. the duration between two menstrual cycles is less than twenty-one days;
2. the bleeding lasts for more than eight days;
3. there is increased blood flow per day irrespective of the duration of menstruation; and
4. you have bleeding six months or more after the last menstruation.

Box 2: Symptoms of menopause

1. Disturbances in menstrual pattern:
   - Absence of ovulation (production of the egg).
   - Reduced fertility.
   - Decreased or increased menstrual flow.
   - Irregular frequency of menstruation.
2. Hot flushes.
3. Psychological symptoms:
   - Anxiety
   - Depression
   - Increased irritability
   - Sleeplessness
   - Decreased sexual desire
4. Decrease in size or functions or a body part (Atrophy):
   - Thinning of the lining of the vagina.
   - Development of small flesh-like projections in the urethra (urethral caruncle).
   - Pain during sexual intercourse.
   - Itching or irritation in the external genital organs.
   - Inability to hold urine, especially while coughing, passing stools, etc.
   - Increased frequency and urgency to pass urine.
   - Inflammation of the urinary tract.

Hot flushes

These are typical and most common symptoms of menopause. During a hot flush, you will have a sudden sensation of warmth or intense heat that spreads over various parts of the body, especially the face, head and chest. Sometimes there may be associated sweating and a feeling of chill. Some women feel very anxious at the time of hot flushes and may have increased heart rate or *palpitations*. Palpitations is the term used for awareness of heart beats that feels like thumping in the chest.

The exact mechanism of development of hot flushes is not yet clear. It is believed that it originates in the brain in response to reduced estrogen levels in the blood. However, not all hot flushes are due to deficiency of estrogen.

Some women believe that hot flushes are due to release of accumulated heat in the body. This is not true. Hot flushes are the result of sudden and abnormal stimulation of the heat release mechanisms in the body. During a hot flush, the skin temperature increases and the conduction capacity of the skin also increases. This is why the body temperature falls at the end of the hot flush. Hot flushes normally last for few seconds to few minutes. The frequency of hot flushes and its duration vary from woman to woman. They are more common at night and during stress.

Box 3 describes the various symptoms associated with a hot flush.

Changes in the structure of the reproductive organs
Estrogen not only plays a very important role in maintaining normal structure and functions of a woman's reproductive organs but also those of the surrounding tissues and organs such as the *urinary bladder* and the *urethra*. When the estrogen level declines after menopause, the tissues of these organs including their inner lining become weak and shrink. Urinary bladder is a muscular bag-like structure that stores urine for discharge through the urethra. Urethra is a small tubular structure that drains urine from the bladder. It opens outside the body just in front of the vagina.

Thinning of the lining of the vagina leads to pain during intercourse and increased dryness. There may also be itching and irritation in the vagina and external genital organs such as the *vulva*. The thinning of vagina and dryness continue to worsen even after menopause. This is why many women have troublesome vaginal irritation and pain during sexual intercourse after the age of fifty-five to sixty years. Regular sexual intercourse can help maintain the moisture and tone of the vagina.

Box 3: Description of a hot flush

Symptom	Description
Sensation	Sudden feeling of heat. May be associated with anxiety.
Heart rate	Increases up to five to thirty-five beats per minute. May have palpitations.
Blood flow to the skin	Increases, which is observed as flushing.
Finger skin temperature	Increases rapidly up to about 1-7ºC. Slowly declines after hot flush ends.
Sweating	Normally profuse and starts suddenly. Drying of sweat depends upon humidity and temperature around you.
Core body temperature	Decreases by about 0.1-0.9ºC several minutes after hot flush starts. Often felt as a chill at the end of the hot flush.
Sleep	Problems in sleeping that increase at night. You may wake up suddenly with hot flush or night sweats.

Thinning and weakening of the urinary bladder increases the risk of urinary infections and pain while passing the urine. It can also lead to involuntary leakage of urine, especially when you cough or sneeze or strain to pass the stools. This is because these actions increase the pressure in the abdomen and push the urine out.

Mood changes

Estrogen plays a very important role in memory and maintaining normal functions of the nerve cells in the brain. This is why some women believe that decreased estrogen levels during menopause cause mood changes, depression and anxiety. However, several psychiatric studies have failed to establish a definite relationship between estrogen levels and emotional disturbances. It is therefore believed that emotional disturbances during menopause may be largely due to various other factors, such as: pressures of career, marriage, increasing demands from growing children, especially adolescents, and responsibilities towards ageing parents.

What is hormone replacement therapy?

Hormone replacement therapy is the term used for supplementation of female sex hormones, especially estrogen, after menopause. The main aim of hormone replacement therapy is to reduce the risk of heart diseases and osteoporosis after menopause and to provide relief from troublesome symptoms of menopause.

Estrogen can be supplemented either daily or in cycles where a few days break is given every month. Progesterone is also added with estrogen in women who have not had hysterectomy. This is to prevent changes in the structure and functions of the inner lining of the uterus. Progesterone supplementation is normally given for ten to fourteen days, depending upon its type. At the end of progesterone supplementation, you will have bleeding, which will be similar to normal menstruation.

Estrogen can be supplemented in three ways:
1. Orally, as tablets;
2. Below the skin, as implants, and
3. Through the skin such as in gel or patch forms.

All the above three ways of estrogen supplementation are effective in management of troublesome symptoms of menopause and protection against bone loss and heart diseases.

In case you have mild symptoms of the urinary system or external genital organs (such as itching, etc.), your doctor is likely to recommend a milder type of estrogen that can be used continuously. You can take it either as tablets or as vaginal cream.

The decisions on when to start hormone replacement therapy and how long to continue it will depend mainly upon your symptoms and assessment of the benefits versus risks of the therapy. The benefits of hormone replacement can start within a few weeks and normally continue as long as you take the replacement. The symptoms can recur when you stop the therapy. This is why most doctors recommend long-term hormone replacement therapy.

Benefits of hormone replacement therapy
Hormone replacement therapy almost always controls hot flushes at night. It also reverses the changes in the structure of the inner lining of the vagina and urinary tract and makes them thick, stimulates vaginal glands to secrete fluids that act as lubrication during sexual intercourse. This is why it can also enhance sexual desire.

Hormone replacement therapy is effective in reducing the risks of heart attack and osteoporosis. These effects are discussed in greater detail in other sections of this book.

Some women report that estrogen helps control their irritability and mood changes. Some studies have indicated that estrogen enhances the effects of medicines used to treat depression.

As age advances, oil production in the glands of the skin reduces. As a result, the skin becomes dry and wrinkled. It is believed that estrogen therapy helps regulate activity of the oil glands in the skin and therefore makes it look younger. It is important to remember that while hormone replacement therapy may improve the skin and hair texture, it is not recommended for this benefit alone.

Risks of hormone replacement therapy

Some studies have indicated that hormone replacement after menopause may increase the risk of breast cancer. However, some other studies have indicated otherwise. They have indicated that the risk of cancer reduces after eight to ten years for estrogen replacement. Since it is not conclusively proven if hormone replacement increases the risk of breast cancer, your doctor will weigh the benefits of protection against heart diseases and osteoporosis with the risk of breast cancer before recommending if you need hormone replacement or not. The relationship between estrogen and breast cancer is discussed in greater detail in subsequent sections of this book.

Estrogen replacement can increase the risk of blood clots in the veins and are therefore not recommended if you have the tendency to develop blood clots in the leg veins.

Some studies have indicated that higher doses of estrogen can worsen high blood pressure. Your doctor will therefore assess the risk of heart attack and then recommend estrogen dose most suited to you.

The benefits and risks associated with hormone replacement therapy are as listed in Box 4.

It is important to remember that there are no common guidelines for hormone replacement therapy that can be applied for all women. The decision is taken on the basis of evaluation of benefits and risks for each woman. Your doctor will assess several factors such as your general health, risk of associated diseases, nutritional status, etc., before deciding on whether or not you are likely to benefit from hormone replacement therapy with little associated risks. *It is strongly recommended that you avoid (a) indiscriminate use of hormones during menopause and (b) practice self medication.*

How are hot flushes managed?

Hot flushes can be managed either by modifying your lifestyle and developing a positive attitude and/or medicines such as hormones and other synthetic preparations.

> **Box 4: Benefits and risks of hormone replacement therapy**
>
> **Benefits:**
> - Relief from symptoms associated with decreased estrogen levels such as hot flushes, vaginal thinning, urinary disturbances, etc.
> - Decreased risk of heart diseases.
> - Decreased risk of osteoporosis and therefore fractures.
> - Increased life expectancy.
> - Decreased risk of cancer of the intestine.
> - Decreased risk of stroke and paralysis.
> - Decreased risk of Alzheimer's disease.
>
> **Risks:**
> - Increased risk of cancer of the inner lining of the uterus, especially if progesterone is not added to the hormone replacement.
> - Increased risk of breast cancer. More studies are needed to determine if hormone replacement increases this risk.
> - Increased risk of blood clots in the veins.

Lifestyle modifications

It is desirable that you make necessary lifestyle adjustments to cope with hot flushes. You first need to identify factors that either increase the frequency of hot flushes or make them more severe. These could be hot drinks, alcohol, caffeine, hot environments, etc. Wear light and loose clothes and avoid heavy foods. Eat large portions of fruits and vegetables. Stress at home and workplace can also worsen hot flushes. You therefore need to practice relaxation techniques such as yoga and meditation to deal with stress effectively.

Deep breathing

Some studies have indicated that deep abdominal breathing can control hot flushes. It is desirable that you breath six to eight times a minute for about fifteen minutes each twice a day.

Exercises

Regular exercises five times a week for at least twenty minutes each time can effectively control hot flushes. Exercises reduce blood levels of some hormones of the brain that influence secretion of estrogen and progesterone by the ovaries. They also increase some chemical substances that decrease during a hot flush.

In case the hot flushes adversely affect your day-to- day work despite attempts to modify factors that aggravate them, you need to consult with your doctor. He/she may recommend hormones to control them. It is important to remember that the available therapies do not cure hot flushes. They provide relief from troublesome symptoms by reducing the frequency of hot flushes and/or making them less intense. Sometimes they may disappear during treatment and recur once you stop the medicines. This is because it is very difficult to predict how long your hot flushes will last and how severe they will be. In order to avoid the hot flushes from recurring when you stop medicines, your doctor is likely to recommend gradual reduction in the dose of medicine over several weeks.

Estrogen

This is the most preferred medicine for management of hot flushes. Its effect is usually not immediate and may take up to several months before the hot flushes are effectively controlled. There are several estrogen preparations and your doctor will prescribe the type of estrogen most suited to you based on your symptoms and other associated health problems, if any. Estrogen can also improve other symptoms such as sleeplessness, dryness in the vagina, lack of memory or concentration, and problems of the urinary tract.

Non-estrogen medicines

Majority of the women get relief from hot flushes with estrogen. In case estrogen is contraindicated for you or you have severe adverse reactions to it, your doctor is likely to recommend medicines that do not contain estrogen, which are called non-estrogen medicines.

Non-estrogen medicines normally recommended for management of hot flushes include progestins and clonidine.

Progestins are mainly of two types: (a) medroxy-progesterone acetate (MPA) and (b) megestrol acetate (MA). MPA can be taken either orally or as injections either in the upper arm or the buttocks. The major side effect of MPA injections is abnormal menstruation. The side effects are relatively less severe when it is taken orally. Hot flushes are normally controlled by the third month of treatment. Oral megestrol acetate or MA has lower risk of abnormal bleeding and depression as compared to MPA. They are therefore preferred for management of hot flushes.

Clonidine, another non-estrogen medicine, is one of the medicines prescribed for control of high blood pressure. It reduces the dilation of blood vessels of the skin, which is commonly associated with hot flushes. Clonidine is especially useful to control hot flushes if you have associated high blood pressure. Its major side effect is dry mouth. Other minor side effects are nausea, headache, fatigue and dizziness.

Vitamin E

Some studies have indicated that taking Vitamin E supplements can reduce the frequency and severity of hot flushes. More studies are however required to determine its effectiveness and the type of people for whom it may be most effective. It is important to remember that indiscriminate use of Vitamin E can harm your body. Since this vitamin is fat-soluble, it accumulates in the body over a period of time. Excessive deposits of any vitamin in the body can adversely affect your health.

What is osteoporosis?

Osteoporosis is defined as a decrease in the bone mass of the body. In other words, the bones become thin. Thinner bones are weak and therefore break easily. This is why various fractures are more common in women after menopause even with minimum injury. Bone loss and weakening is natural with age and occurs in men also. It, however, occurs more rapidly in women after menopause. Box 5 lists the proposed risk factors for osteoporosis.

Box 5: Proposed risk factors of osteoporosis

- **Hereditary:** Sex, race, history of osteoporosis in other family members.
- **Nutritional:** Low calcium intake, high intake of alcohol, caffeine, salt or proteins, especially animal protein.
- **Lifestyle:** Smoking and sedentary lifestyle.
- **Hormones:** Decreased activity of the ovaries and body composition.
- **Diseases:** Increased activity of the parathyroid or thyroid glands, defective absorption of some nutrients, liver diseases, excess of a chemical substance called glucocorticoid and surgical removal of part of the stomach.

Symptoms

Unless there is fracture, osteoporosis normally does not cause any symptoms. Fractures due to osteoporosis are more common in the backbone, wrist, hip, upper part of the hand and pelvis.

Diagnosis

It is easy to diagnose osteoporosis in older women who have a fracture. Normally blood tests to measure the levels of calcium, phosphorus and alkaline phosphatase are recommended to rule out other associated diseases of the bones. In case your doctor suspects some disorders of other organs of the body (listed in Box 4), he/she is likely to recommend further tests to make an accurate diagnosis.

Bone mass measurement

Several newer techniques are now available that can accurately assess bone mass as compared to a conventional x-ray. These include *single and dual photon absorptiometry* and *CT scanning*. Photon is the smallest quantity of electromagnetic energy. It can occur in the form of x-rays, gamma rays or a quantum of light. Single and dual photon absorptiometry is the procedure where the amount of photon received by the bones is measured. The results indicate the density of the bone mass. CT scanning or computed tomography is an x-ray technique that produces films representing detailed cut sections of the bones. It is a painless and non-invasive procedure and therefore requires no special preparation before the test.

Several studies have indicated that measurement of bone mass can assess the future risk of fractures. Depending on the results of bone mass assessment, your doctor will be able to decide whether you require hormone replacement therapy or not to reduce the risk of osteoporosis.

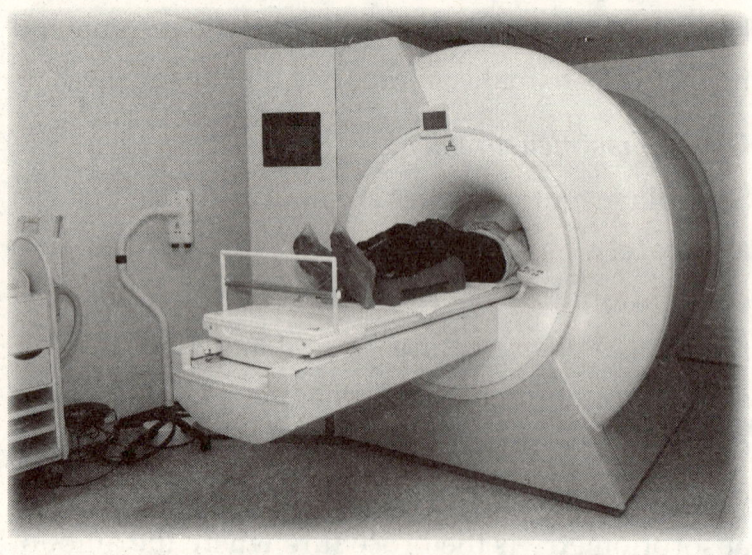

Treatment

After confirming diagnosis of a fracture due to osteoporosis, your doctor will recommend rest, painkillers and other medicines to relax the muscles. Immobilisation of the affected part of the body is avoided as far as possible because lack of movement itself can lead to bone loss.

The pain normally subsides within a few weeks provided no fresh fractures occur. Your doctor is also likely to recommend calcium tablets and estrogen replacement therapy, provided you are below sixty-five years of age and do not have any contraindication for taking estrogen.

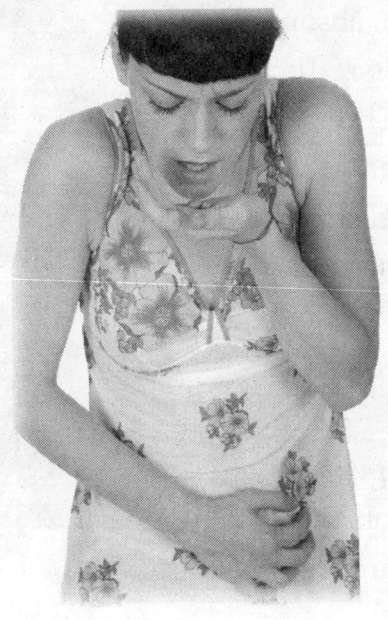

Prevention

The best way to reduce the risk of osteoporosis and associated fractures is to prevent bone loss. There are several preventive measures to reduce the risks, and each is believed to have a role. You need to start these preventive measures early, at least just before or during menopause, in order to ensure that they are effective. You can prevent osteoporosis through the following methods:

Calcium intake

Several studies have persuasively indicated that inadequate calcium intake adversely affects the bones in the body. Calcium absorption from the intestines reduce as age advances. Thus, calcium deficiency gets worse when you do not consume adequate calcium in the diet, which will be more than your earlier requirement.

In order to prevent osteoporosis, you need to consume about eight hundred to fifteen hundred milligrams of calcium per day. Most medical researchers opine that the type of calcium you take — whether in your diet or as supplement — is not important. However, more studies are needed to establish the most effective way to ensure adequate calcium intake by the body. It is desirable that you develop a dietary pattern that includes larger portions of calcium rich foods. Rich sources of calcium commonly available in the Indian diet include cereals such as ragi, milk and milk products, and fruits such as custard apple.

Exercise

Prolonged periods of immobilisation of the body leads to increased bone loss. It is believed that moderate and regular exercises reduce the bone loss in older age groups.

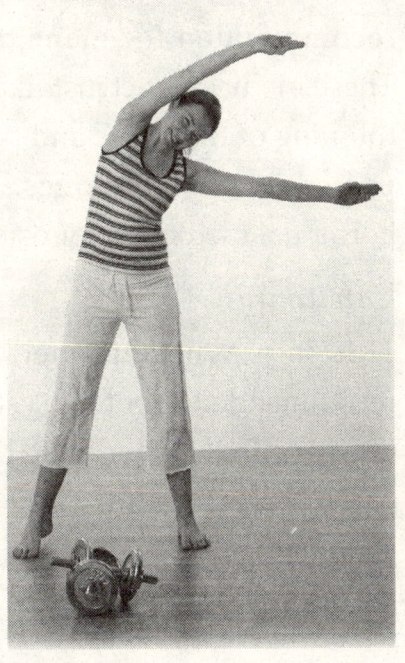

Estrogen

The most effective way to prevent bone loss in women during and after menopause is to take estrogen. The minimum effective dose of estrogen depends upon the type of estrogen, calcium intake and other associated factors that increase the risk of bone loss. Most women need to continue estrogen therapy for about five to ten years.

As mentioned earlier, estrogen therapy can cause several side effects. Your doctor will therefore first assess the risk of osteoporosis and then recommend estrogen, if necessary.

Non-hormonal medicines for osteoporosis

Sometimes medicines other than estrogen are recommended for management of osteoporosis. These medicines act just like estrogen. They prevent thinning of the bones and prevent calcium for being pulled out of the bones. Commonly used non-hormonal medicines for osteoporosis include:

Calcitonin

This is a synthetic medicine that is normally recommended about five years after menopause. It is effective for women who have already developed osteoporosis and for whom estrogen is contraindicated.

Selective estrogen receptor modulators

This medicine is recommended for women who do not have hot flushes but are at risk of developing osteoporosis. It is not recommended if you have hot flushes as they can worsen them. It is also not recommended if you are at risk of developing blood clots in the veins or have liver disease.

Blophosphonates

This medicine reduces the activities of cells that induce bone loss. Blophosphonates have several side effects and are therefore not routinely recommended.

What is the effect of menopause on heart diseases?

The risk of heart diseases rapidly increases in women after menopause. The risk is more if you have one or more of the following associated risk factors:

- Obesity
- High blood pressure
- Cigarette smoking
- Sedentary lifestyle
- High levels of bad cholesterol in the blood
- Diabetes

As mentioned earlier, the levels of estrogen and progesterone are different before puberty, during reproductive age and after menopause. These changes in the hormone levels affect different organs of the body such as the heart and blood vessels in different ways. Some of these effects can either reduce or increase the risk of heart diseases.

What is the effect of oral contraceptive pills on heart diseases?

There has been a lot of debate on whether the use of oral contraceptive pills increases the risk of stroke and heart attacks in women. When oral contraceptive pills were first manufactured, more than thirty years ago, they contained very high doses of estrogen, which was attributed to the increased risk of heart attacks and strokes. However, recent preparations of oral contraceptive pills contain about one-third of the original dose of estrogen. Also, the recent pills have derivatives of progesterone, which lower the blood levels of bad cholesterol and increase the level of good cholesterol. They, therefore, reduce the risk of heart diseases, especially heart attack. Some studies have, however, indicated that the newer derivatives of progesterone can increase the risk of blood clots in the veins of the legs.

The risk of heart attack because of oral contraceptives is higher in women above thirty-five years of age, who have high blood pressure and who are smokers. This risk is not associated with the dose of hormones in the pills or the duration of their use. After the pills are stopped, the risk reduces. The risk of heart attack due to oral contraceptive pills is lower in women below thirty-five years of age.

Although most medical practitioners opine that the overall risk-benefit ratio for risk of heart attack and oral contraceptives is low in women who do not smoke, it is important that you consult your doctor before starting oral contraceptive pills.

What is the effect of estrogen on heart diseases?
Several studies have indicated that women who use estrogen after menopause are at lower risk of heart diseases as compared to those who do not use them. Box 6 lists the various mechanisms by which estrogen protects the heart.

Some studies have indicated that although estrogen replacement therapy after menopause reduces the risk of heart attack, it may increase the risk of other diseases such as breast cancer and blood clots in the veins. As mentioned earlier, your doctor will decide whether the benefits of estrogen

Box 6: Protective mechanism of estrogen on the heart

- Favourably altering fats in the blood.
- Increase blood levels of good cholesterol.
- Decrease blood levels of bad cholesterol.
- Effects on the reactivity of the blood vessels.
- Antioxidant effects, which means inhibition or retardation of oxidation. Oxidation is the process by which oxygen is added to a substance. Estrogen inhibits oxidation of bad cholesterol.
- Changes in fibrinogen — a protein in the blood that is essential for clotting of blood.
- Direct effect on the cells and blood vessels of the heart which improves the pumping action of the heart.
- Reduce abnormal multiplication of the cells of the heart muscles.
- Improves overall functions of the pancreas and therefore decreases insulin and glucose levels.
- Action on other hormones that may have direct or indirect relationship to atherosclerosis (hardening and thickening of blood vessels).

replacement are more than the expected risks before recommending hormone replacement therapy. There are several types of hormone preparations available. Based on your other associated risk factors and general health, your doctor will be able to recommend the most suited preventive measure for major diseases.

What is the effect of estrogen on breast cancer?

Several studies have indicated that female sex hormones influence development of breast cancer in all stages. All preventive measures to reduce the risk of breast cancer are based on the following understanding of the relationship of these hormones to the risk of breast cancer:

1. Early menopause reduces the risk of breast cancer. Women who have menopause after the age of fifty years are at greater risk of breast cancer.

2. Early onset of menstruation (menarche), especially before eleven years of age, increases the risk of breast cancer.

3. Estrogen replacement therapy after menopause increases the risk of breast cancer to a relatively small extent.

4. Obesity after menopause increases the risk of breast cancer. However, obesity before menopause marginally reduces the risk of breast cancer.
5. Oral contraceptive pills do not decrease the risk of breast cancer.

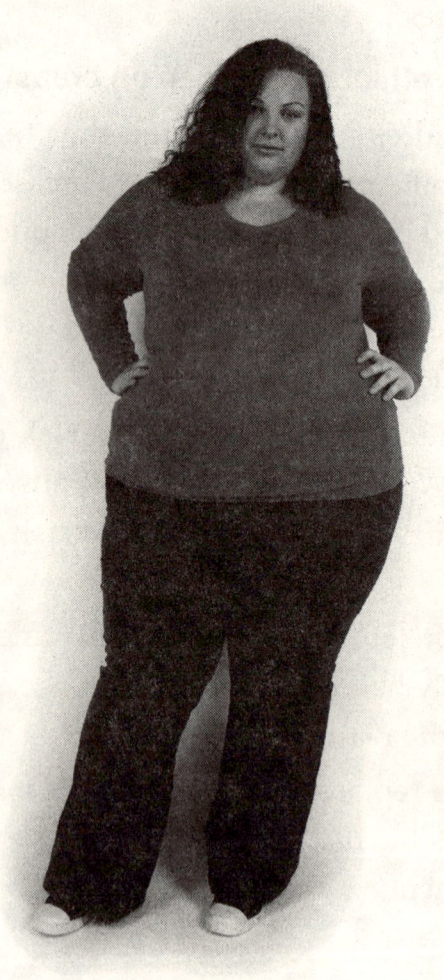

Family history is very important in establishing risk levels for breast cancer. Immediate blood relatives of women who have had breast cancer have a two to three times higher risk of developing breast cancer. Cancers of ovary and uterus also increase the risk.

Many women are concerned with the effect of estrogen replacement therapy on the breast. This is mainly because of the risk associated with oral contraceptive pills and breast cancer. The level of estrogen in most birth control pills is much higher than the dose recommended for replacement therapy. This is why, you should not worry about developing breast cancer if your doctor recommends hormone replacement therapy.

He/she will, however, not recommend this therapy if you have other risks of developing breast cancer, such as breast cancer in your immediate blood relatives, etc.

What is the effect of menopause on sexual desire?

Many women report decreased sexual desire after menopause. Box 7 lists the factors that influence sexual behaviour among older women.

Hormone replacement therapy is often effective in enhancing sexual desire. In case you have pain during sexual act because there is not enough lubrication in the vagina, you can adopt several ways to ensure painless sexual intercourse. Regular sexual activity is one of the effective ways to maintain moisture of the vagina. Having bath with warm water before intercourse, and using lubricants such as K-Y jelly can relieve pain during sex.

Box 7: Factors influencing sexual behaviour in older women

Changes in the structure of reproductive organs:
- Decrease in size of the vagina.
- Thinning of walls of the vagina.
- Poor lubrication inside vagina.
- Decreased blood flow to the vagina.
- Decreased sensitivity in the vagina.
- Decreased size of the external genital organs.
- Inflammation or infections of the vagina.

Changes in the structure of the breast:
- Reduced size of the breast.
- Reduced "swelling" of the breast during sexual arousal.
- Altered touch sensation of the nipples and the area around it.

Changes in the structure of pelvis:
- Reduced tone of the muscles around the vagina.

Hormonal changes:
- Decreased estrogen and progesterone levels in blood.
- Increased blood level of some hormones secreted by the brain that influence secretion of estrogen and progesterone.

Major diseases:
- Diabetes.
- Heart diseases such as congestive heart failure and angina.
- Arthritis.
- Cancer.
- Surgery of reproductive organs such as hysterectomy, etc.
- Dementia.

Use of medicines:
- Regular alcohol intake.
- Some medicines used to control high blood pressure.

Psychological factors:
- Increased risk of anxiety and depression.
- Lack of sexual partner.
- Negative attitudes of society towards sexuality in older women.
- Religious beliefs.
- Lack of privacy such as due to living with children or in smaller homes.

Ayurveda

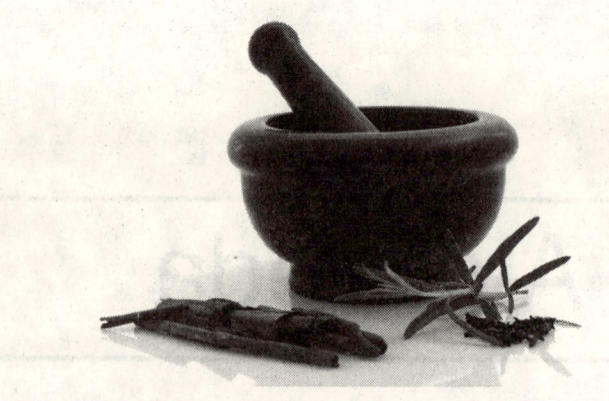

Ayurveda also describes menopause as a condition when menstruation stops due to decline in activities of the ovaries. It is mentioned in several ancient literatures as *Vigatartava* or *Nishphala*. Sushruta, the ancient Ayurvedic surgeon, describes the initial stage of menstruation at twelve years of age, which is the age of menarche, and end of menstruation at about fifty years. This climacteric change is attributed to factors such as ageing and over-maturity of the female body constituents at an advanced age. Other Ayurvedic scholars such as Kashyapa, Vagabhatta, Acharya Bhavamishra and Arunadatta have also agreed with the same description.

Charaka, a famous ancient Ayurvedic physician, opines that no disease or disorder inside the human body can be precipitated without the imbalance of the three doshas: *vata*, *pitta* and *kapha*. Competent Ayurvedic physicians treat various health problems or diseases by first assessing the imbalance of the three doshas and then prescribe medicines that are most appropriate to restore the normal balance of these doshas. This is why it is not necessary to name all diseases or health problems.

Maharshi Bhela, an Ayurvedic seer, has stated that menstruation is a sign of maturity of the *Dhatus* (body constituents) such as *Rasa* (plasma), *Rakta* (blood), *Mansa* (muscle), *Meda* (fat tissue), *Asthi* (bone), *Majja* (mucous) and *Shukra* (sperm). The secondary sex changes also occur in boys and girls normally after twelve years of age due to the maturity of *dhatus* or body constituents. In girls, these changes are growth of superficial hair in the underarms and pubic region, development of breasts and onset of menstruation. During this stage, there is also a gradual development of reproductive organs such as uterus, vagina and vulva. This entire process reverses during menopause or *Nishpala* stage of women around fifty years of age. This is why there is degradation of various parts of the body and organs of the reproductive system. This degradation adversely affects the physical, metabolic, digestive, hormonal and psychosexual behaviour of women. In addition to cessation of menstruation, there is increased risk of loss of density of the bones, heart diseases, problems of the urinary system and degenerative changes of the skin.

How is menopause managed?

Management of symptoms of menopause is mainly *Yukti Vipashreya* (use of therapeutic measures) and *Satwavajaya* (psychotherapy). Satwavajaya helps you to understand the changes taking place in your body and therefore prepares you mentally to deal with them effectively. It will also clarify all your doubts, misconceptions and therefore remove fears associated with menopause. Detailed below are the medicines commonly recommended for management of troublesome symptoms of menopause.

Single medicines recommended for management of troublesome symptoms of menopause include:
- *Ashwagandha (Withania somnifetra) Ksirapaka:* Boil ten grams of the Ashwagandha (Winter cherry) powder with two hundred and fifty millilitres each of milk and water at medium temperature. Keep on boiling it till the total volume reduces to half. Add two teaspoon of sugar and take this medicine once a day, preferably before noon.

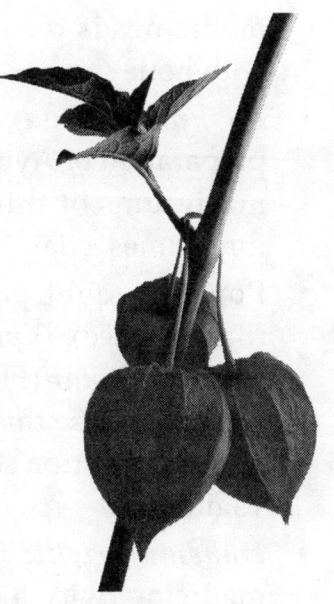

- Three to five grams of powdered *Shankhapushpa* (butterfly pea) or *Sarpagandha* (Rauwolfia serpentina) or *Brahmi* (Thyme leaved gratiola) to be taken twice a day with water.

Simple and compound preparations recommended for management of troublesome symptoms of menopause include:
- *Pushyaguna powder:* Take two to thee grams of this powder twice a day with honey followed by two hundred millilitres of clean water used to

wash rice. This water contains starch, which enhances the effects of the medicine.
- ***Rajatidoshahara Vati, Somnanath Rasa, Pradaranlaki Lauha, Shilajatwadi Lauha***: Two hundred and fifty milligrams of each of these medicines is recommended three times a day with honey.
- ***Pushpadhanwa Rasa***: This is a classical preparation of Ayurveda. Two hundred and fifty milligrams of this medicine is recommended three times a day.
- Powder equal portions of the bark of ***Vata*** (Banyan tree), ***Pipal*** (Sacred fig), ***Gular*** (Cluster fig) and ***Pakar*** (Ficus infectoria) and prepare a decoction. Use this decoction as vaginal douche and insert cotton soaked in ***Jatyadi*** oil inside the vagina.
- ***Dahsmularisht:*** Take thirty millilitres of this medicine twice a day, i.e., one hour after each meal. You need to take this medicine with equal volume of water.
- Proprietary preparations such as Genifort, Vigoron, M-2 Ton (Charaka) Vigorex, Fortige (Alarsan) are some of the commercial preparations recommended for management of troublesome symptoms of menopause.
- ***Bala Tail:*** This can be used as *sonehava/abhyanga* every day or at least on alternate days.

What are the dietary and lifestyle recommendations during menopause?

Ayurveda recommends that you eat simple and easily digestible foods, especially fruits. Take adequate rest, and do light exercises in the open air regularly. There are few specific yogasanas that you need to learn from a yoga expert and practice them regularly. In addition, take precautions to avoid constipation and maintain regular bowel movements.

Homoeopathy

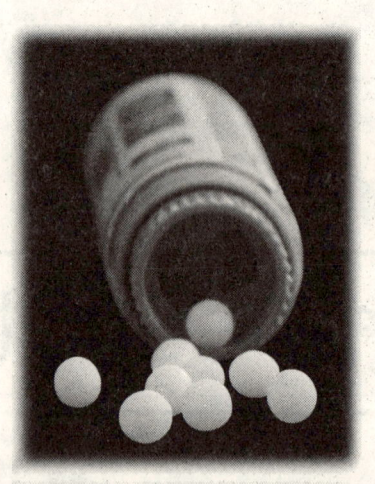

The causes, signs, symptoms and risks of menopause as per Homoeopathy are the same as those detailed in the section on Allopathy.

What is the aim of Homoeopathic management of menopause?

Homoeopathic medicines act on the "vital force" of the body to provide a dynamic stimulus that restores the delicate balance of the various hormones in your body. These medicines thus treat your entire body rather than just the reproductive organs. They also enhance your body's natural defence mechanism and restore your health to optimum. Homoeopathy does not recommend hormones for management of menopause.

What is the mechanism of action of Homoeopathic medicines recommended for menopause?

Homoeopathic medicines recommended for menopause have two main actions: (a) providing quick relief to the physical and mental problems; and (b) eradicating the negative effects or reduced effects of estrogen on various parts of the body such as bones, joints, heart, etc.

What is the Homoeopathic approach to management of menopause?

Just as for all other conditions, your physician will take a detailed history.

He/she will especially focus on:
- Your present symptoms, their severity and factors that worsen them;
- Any health problems in the past, with special emphasis on any unusual physical or mental trauma just prior to the onset of menopause;
- Past frequency of menstrual cycles, its duration, associated symptoms, etc.;
- Number of pregnancies, their outcome and problems, if any, during pregnancy or delivery;
- Specific health problems in your family;
- Your likes, dislikes, habits, etc.; and
- Your mental make-up.

Your physician may also recommend various tests such as blood tests, urine tests, pap smear, etc., to eliminate the possibility of serious health problems.

How is menopause managed?

Detailed below are some of the Homoeopathic medicines used more commonly for management of menopause:

Lachesis

This is one of the most commonly used medicines for management of menopause. It is normally recommended for women who have hot flushes, suffocated feeling especially during sleep, aversion to any tight clothing around the neck, preference of open air. Such women are often talkative and suspicious by nature.

Graphites
This medicine is normally recommended for fat women of about forty to fifty years of age who have had menstrual irregularities. It is especially recommended for women who have constipation, feel sensitive to cold and have unhealthy skin.

Sepia
This is a very effective medicine for correction of hormonal imbalances and its adverse effects. It is especially recommended for women who are tall, thin, have masculine features, are emotionally closed, and often indifferent to their loved ones. Such women are also short-tempered, aggressive and have a marked aversion to sexual activities. They often have abnormal white discharge from the vagina.

Natrum Mur
This medicine is recommended for women who have suffered from grief or emotional trauma before the onset of symptoms of menopause. It is especially effective for women who have scanty, irregular menstruation, hot flushes, severe headache on exposure to sun. Most women with these symptoms have depression and prefer solitude. They also crave excess salt in their food.

Ignatia

This medicine is recommended for women who had severe shock and are therefore withdrawn and quiet. It is especially effective for women who have a tendency to become hysterical.

Calcarea Carb

This medicine is recommended for obese women with a tendency for constipation, who have joint pains that worsens with exposure to cold or damp weather. It is especially effective for women who have excessive craving for eggs, who have scanty or excessive menstruation, excessive white discharge from vagina, backache and joint pains.

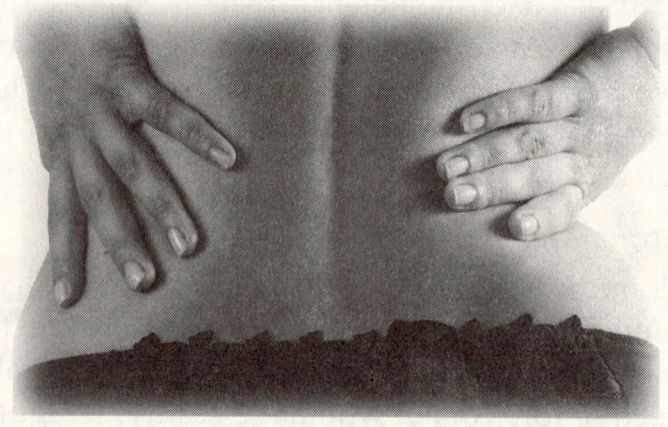

There are several other Homoeopathic medicines that are effective in treating various symptoms of menopause. Your doctor will select the medicine most suited to you on the basis of the totality of your symptoms.

Homoeopathy strongly recommends general measures also for management of menopause. These include:
- Regular exercise to maintain normal weight for your height and age, and to ensure that your bones and joints are healthy and mobile.
- A diet rich in calcium and other minerals and vitamins. You need to eat larger portions of vegetables, fruits, milk, cheese, etc., and take smaller portions of fat. It is desirable that you avoid red meat and foods that are rich in cholesterol.
- Practice relaxation techniques such as yoga, meditation, breathing exercises, etc., to avoid stress and maintain normal mental health.
- Keep yourself involved in activities that keep you emotionally satisfied and cheerful. This will help avoid stress and loneliness.

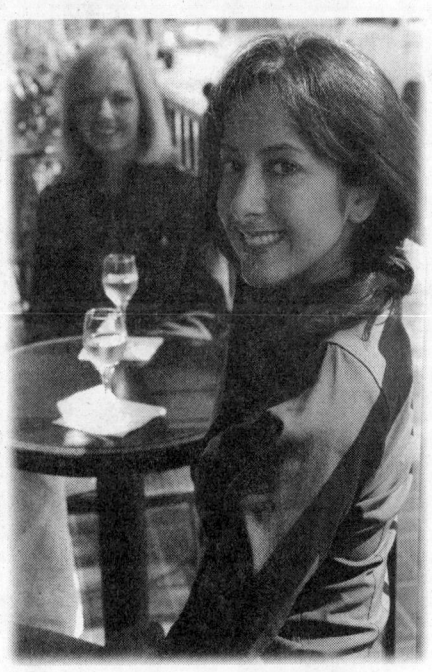

- Maintain good personal hygiene to prevent infections, especially those of the genital area.

It is important to remember that indiscriminate use of Homoeopathic medicines without direct supervision of a doctor can cause adverse effects.

Nature Cure

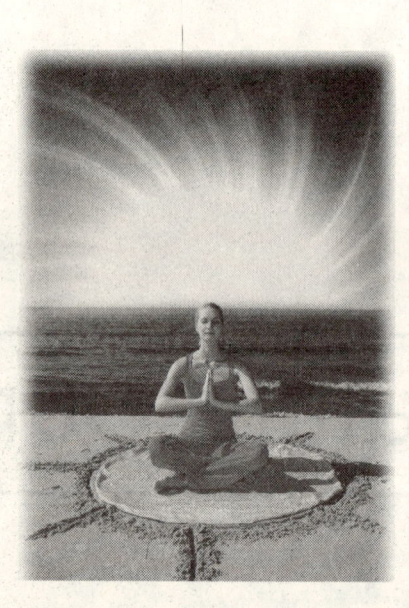

Definition, types, signs and symptoms of menopause as per Nature Cure system of medicine are the same as those detailed in the section on Allopathy.

How is menopause managed?

According to Nature Cure, a large number of women experience increased volume and/or longer duration of menstruation during menopause, which leads to anaemia and general weakness. The priority should be given to control excessive bleeding during menopause. In case there is normal bleeding per day but the menstruation lasts for a longer duration, you need to adopt treatment measures to control menstruation after three days of bleeding.

Nature Cure recommends the following measures for controlling excessive menstruation.

Ice cold compress

Dip a cotton cloth in ice cold water and apply it to the pubic region every hour for ten to fifteen minutes each time until menstruation stops.

Mud packs

Prepare a mud pack preferably in ice cold water and apply it to the pubic region every hour for ten to fifteen minutes each time.

Cold foot bath

Immerse both legs up to calf muscles in a bucket of cold water for five to seven minutes each three times a day. You can add ice cubes in the water for enhanced effect.

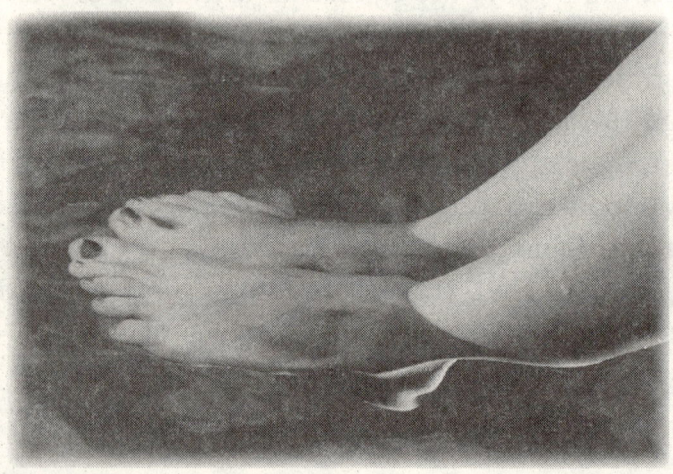

Cold douche

Take cold douche for the lower part of the back for three to four minutes each time about two to three times a day till bleeding stops.

Hip bath

After the bleeding stops, you need to take hip bath twice a day for fifteen minutes each. Hip bath is like a tonic for the lower abdomen and helps maintain normal functions of the ovaries and a regular menstrual cycle.

According to Nature Cure, most symptoms of menopause such as hot flushes, palpitation, anxiety, depression, mood swings, sleep disturbances, decreased sexual desire and increased sweating at nights are due to irritation of the nervous system. It recommends the following management options to reduce irritation of the nervous system:

Cold spinal bath

A special tub is used for spinal bath in which columns of cold water are passed on the back in such a way that it touches only the backbone. Cold spinal bath reduces the irritation of the nerves. You need to take cold spinal bath for twenty to thirty minutes twice a day and continue it till the symptoms subside.

In case you do not have access to spinal bath tub, you can use a long turkey towel. Fold the towel lengthwise and dip it in cold water. Lie down on your abdomen and apply the cold towel on the backbone. Another alternative to cold spinal bath is to sit on a stool and direct a stream of cold water from a hose-pipe attached to a tap. Do not put water on other parts of the body.

Mud bath

Applying mud on the entire body for one hour every week helps relieve most of the troublesome symptoms of menopause.

Oil massage

Smear oil on the entire body and knead the body parts. This type of massage is also effective in reducing the severity of symptoms associated with menopause.

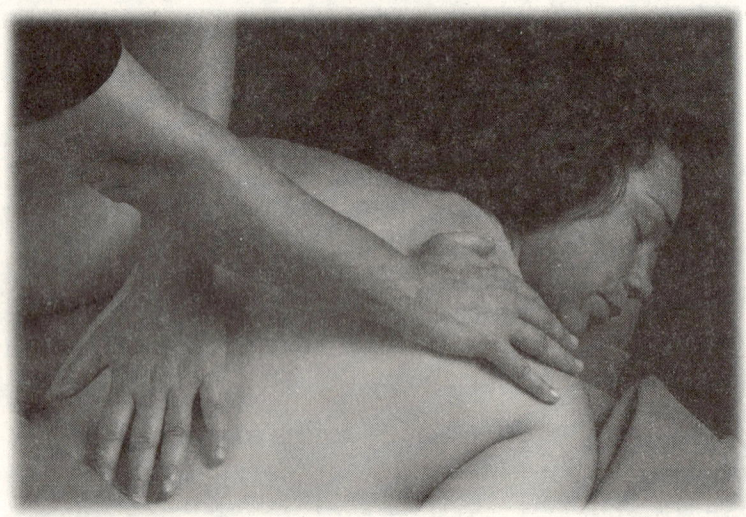

Wet girdle pack

This pack should be used at bed time only. To wear this pack, you need to use two cotton underwears that fit you tightly. Dip the first underwear in cold water, squeeze it to remove excess water and wear it on bare skin. Wear the second dry underwear on the wet underwear. You can then wear your normal night dress and go to sleep. Wear the wet girdle pack for the entire night. Wet girdle pack strengthens the muscles of the uterus and helps control excessive bleeding.

Sun bath

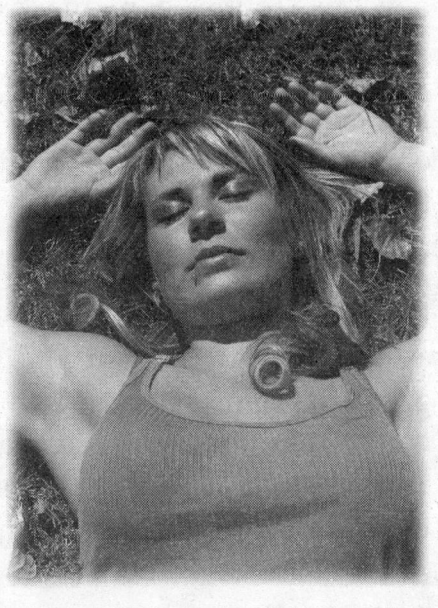

Nature Cure recommends sun bath every day for twenty minutes either before 9.00 a.m. or after 4.00 p.m. in order to prevent loss of bone density. Sunlight will help your skin absorb Vitamin D, which is essential for calcium metabolism in the body.

What are the dietary recommendations during menopause?

Obesity, calcium deficiency, anaemia and other nutritional deficiencies are more common among women during menopause. Nature Cure recommends the following dietary modifications during menopause.

Total calorie intake

In order to control your weight, you need to reduce intake of fats and eat larger portions of vegetables and fruits. In case you are obese, you need to moderate intake of cereals also. Diet alone is not very effective in controlling excessive weight. You need to develop a routine of regular exercises.

Fasting

It is desirable that you fast once a week on liquids only in order to control weight and ensure effective functioning of the digestive system.

Vegetables

Increase your intake of cruciferous vegetables such as broccoli, brussels sprouts, cabbage, cauliflower, green soft mustard, turnip greens, radish, watercress, etc., because they contain protective factors such as *indoles*. These protective factors increase the production of some enzymes that help reduce the adverse effects of reduced female hormones during menopause.

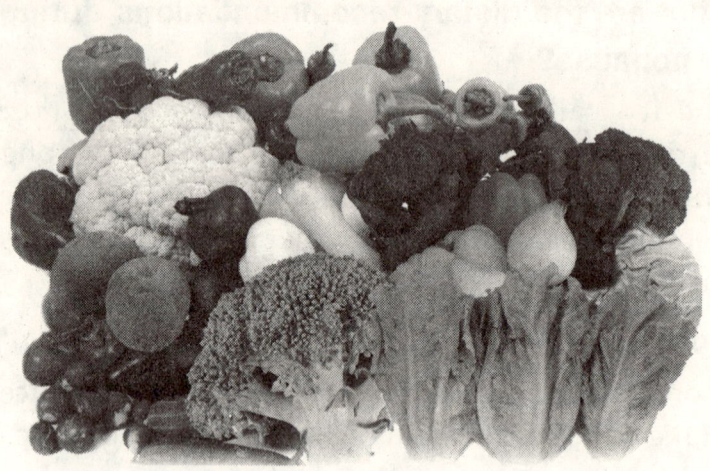

Vitamins

You need to increase intake of fruits, vegetables and milk in order to prevent deficiencies of Vitamins D and E and calcium.

Avoid intake of alcohol, coffee, tea and smoking. Coffee and tea increase the excretion of calcium from the body and therefore increase the risk of loss of bone density.

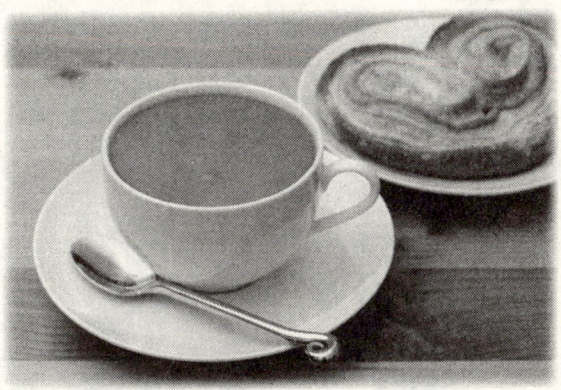

Reduce iron intake

According to Nature Cure, iron tends to accumulate in women after menopause. This is because there is no loss of iron in the menstrual flow. In order to prevent adverse effects of excessive iron deposits in the body, you need to avoid, or reduce intake of animal sources of iron, especially meat. Plant sources of iron such as green leafy vegetables, grains and beans are absorbed less than the animal sources of iron. This is why you can continue to eat all vegetables, grains and beans.

Wild yam

Tincture of wild yam helps prevent osteoporosis and maintain normal balance of female sex hormones.

In addition to the above management options, Nature Cure strongly recommends regular outdoor exercises such as walking, etc., and practice of relaxation techniques such as yoga and meditation in order to control troublesome symptoms of menopause.

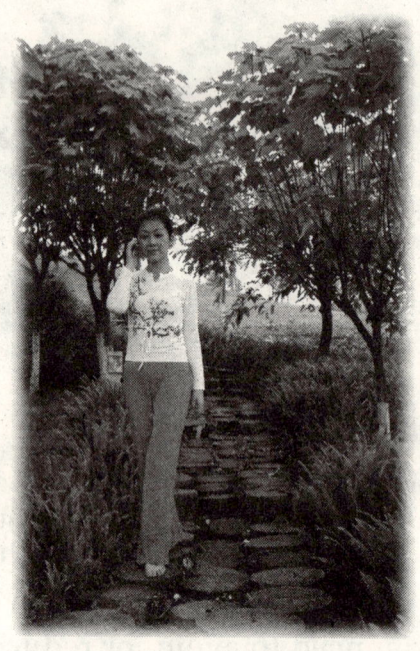

Unani

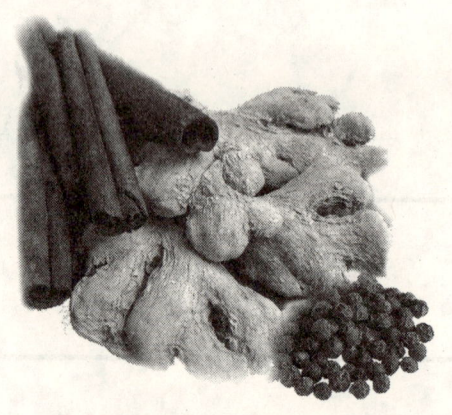

Menopause is known as *Sin-e-yass* in the Unani system of medicine. The symptoms of menopause as per the Unani system of medicine are the same as those listed in the section on Allopathy.

According to the Unani system of medicine, the human life can be divided into three phases. These include (a) *Sin-e-Namu*, in which the body gains are more than the losses; (b) *Sin-e-Balughat*, in which the body gains are equal to the losses; and (c) *Sin-e-Yass*, in which the body gains are less than the losses and the body tissues begin to deteriorate gradually. Menopause indicates one of the physiological degeneration of the female genital organs. The symptoms that a woman experiences because of inactivity of the ovaries are collectively called *Sin-e-yass*. They are at a peak during the first two to three years of menopause and then gradually decrease.

The temperament of women changes during *Sin-e-yass*. This is because *Ratubat-e-badan* are reduced in this phase. This is why Unani physicians recommend diet that has more water content.

How is menopause managed?

Management of menopause is based on the symptoms and aim to restore the altered temperament to normal. *Barid* and *Ratab* medicines are normally effective in these cases.

Single medicines recommended for management of menopause include Asgandh,

Gulnar, Balchar, Amla, Annesoon, Suddab, Karafs, Sandal, Kishneez, Tabasher, Gaozuban, Anjeer and Pista.

Compound medicines recommended for management of menopause include Jawarish Shahi, Jawarish Mastagi, Khamira Abresham, Khamira Gaozuban Ambari Ood Salib wala, Jawarish Anarain, Muraba Amla, Muraba Kalela, Bawaul Misk and Khamira Marwareed.

The dose and duration of treatment with any of the above medicines will depend on your symptoms. Your physician is therefore the best person to recommend the type of medicine along with its most appropriate dose.

Herbal Extracts

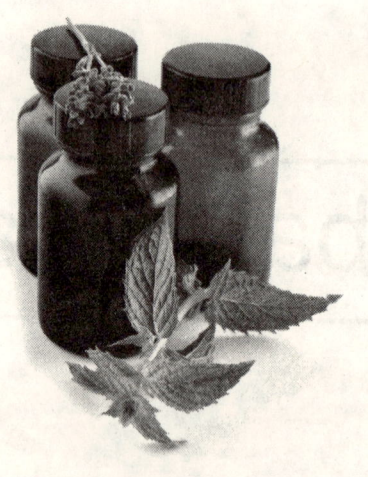

Several herbal extracts have been reported to be effective for management of menstrual problems, including menopause. Of these, Evening Primrose Oil is very widely used, especially for control of hot flushes. This oil is extracted from the seeds of the Evening Primrose flower. This flower is yellow in colour and blooms between six and seven in the evening. The extracted oil is clear, pale yellow in appearance. It does not contain any artificial colour or additives.

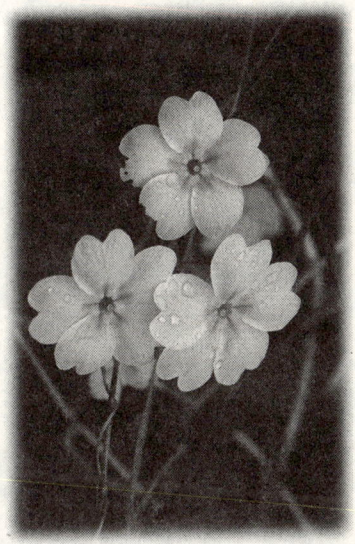

What are the benefits of Evening Primrose Oil?

Evening Primrose Oil has two main benefits: (a) relieve menstrual problems and (b) maintain healthy skin. In addition, the oil also helps prevent brittle nails, dry eyes and dry mouth and helps maintain healthy hair.

Effects on the skin

Evening Primrose Oil helps to make the skin smooth, prevent dryness and reduce excessive loss of water. Some studies have also indicated that the oil may also help slow down the ageing process. These benefits are observed irrespective of whether you take the oil orally as capsules or apply it on the skin.

Menstrual problems

Evening Primrose Oil reduces the adverse impacts of premenstrual syndrome. This is a condition in which some women have one or more of a wide range of symptoms such as nervousness, irritability, emotional disturbances, depression, pain in the

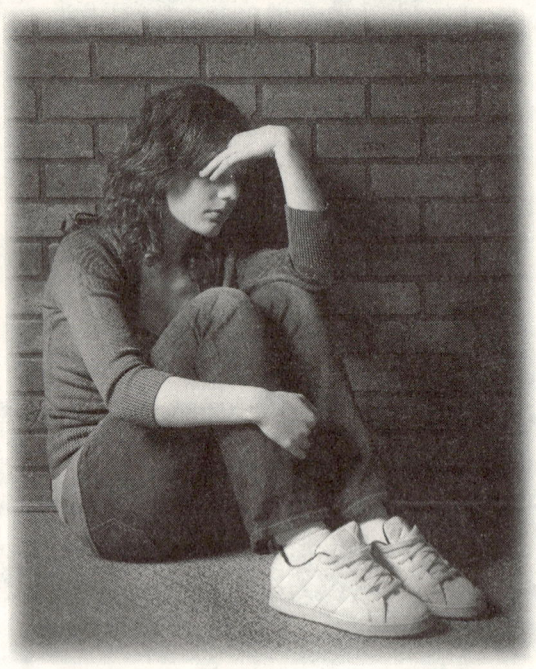

breasts, bloating sensation, headache, nausea, pimples on the face, fatigue, etc. They begin up to ten days before the beginning of menstruation and normally disappear when menstruation starts. Sometimes they may continue for up to two days after menstruation starts.

How does Evening Primrose Oil act?

The benefits of Evening Primrose Oil are because of two *essential fatty acids*. Fatty acids are the basic units of fats. Some fatty acids are synthesised in the body while some others need to be obtained from the diet. Fatty acids that are obtained from the diet are called essential fatty acids. Reduced level of essential fatty acids can lead to an apparent excess of a female hormone called "prolactin". Evening Primrose Oil helps reduce the adverse effects of such chemical imbalances in the body during a woman's menstrual cycle.

There are two types of fatty acids in Evening Primrose Oil — linoleic acid and gamma-linoleic acid (GLA). Women who have menstrual problems are thought to have lower levels of essential fatty acids and *prostaglandin E1*. Prostaglandin is one of a group of hormone like substances present in a wide range of body tissues and fluids including the uterus. One of the actions of prostaglandin is to cause contraction of the uterus. Evening Primrose Oil also contains prostaglandin.

Evening Primrose Oil is not a medicine but a food supplement and does not have any known side effects.

How should Evening Primrose Oil be taken?

Depending upon the severity of your symptoms, you need to take two to four capsules of Evening Primrose Oil seven days before the expected date for menstruation and continued till three days after menstruation starts.

Several commercial preparations of Evening Primrose Oil are available in India, such as *Sunova Efarelle*.